Maria Helena Ferrari
Luciano Duarte Souza

The influence of tomato by-products on feed for Japanese quails

Maria Helena Ferrari
Luciano Duarte Souza

The influence of tomato by-products on feed for Japanese quails

On egg quality

ScienciaScripts

Imprint
Any brand names and product names mentioned in this book are subject to trademark, brand or patent protection and are trademarks or registered trademarks of their respective holders. The use of brand names, product names, common names, trade names, product descriptions etc. even without a particular marking in this work is in no way to be construed to mean that such names may be regarded as unrestricted in respect of trademark and brand protection legislation and could thus be used by anyone.

Cover image: www.ingimage.com

This book is a translation from the original published under ISBN 978-3-330-76719-5.

Publisher:
Sciencia Scripts
is a trademark of
Dodo Books Indian Ocean Ltd. and OmniScriptum S.R.L publishing group

120 High Road, East Finchley, London, N2 9ED, United Kingdom
Str. Armeneasca 28/1, office 1, Chisinau MD-2012, Republic of Moldova, Europe
Managing Directors: Ieva Konstantinova, Victoria Ursu
info@omniscriptum.com

Printed at: see last page
ISBN: 978-620-8-56689-0

DEDICATORY

To my parents, Valdir Lino de Souza and Irani Duarte Souza, for their affection and dedication to the family, for their examples and for their efforts in my personal and professional development, and to all those who incessantly seek knowledge through new technologies.

ACKNOWLEDGEMENTS

To God, first of all, for my life and for granting me another stage in my journey and for the joy he gives me every day.

(There were many people who collaborated in this work and helped to complete it).

To my parents, Valdir and Irani, for their support.

To my supervisor, Professor Márcia Izumi Sakamoto, for her patience and understanding in times of difficulty.

To my professors at the Postgraduate Programme in Animal Production and to all the collaborators in the experimental part who made this work possible.

To Predilecta, for donating the tomato waste used in this study.

Finally, to everyone who, directly or indirectly, contributed to the realisation of this work, thank you very much.

PRESENTATION

Nowadays, there is a growing mobilisation of people interested in issues related to environmental problems. As a result, every processing industry or agro-industry has to be concerned about the rational disposal of its waste.

The increase in ecological awareness that began at the end of the 20th century has made it clear that humanity's great challenge for the coming decades is to balance the production of goods and services, economic growth, social equality and environmental sustainability.

In Latin America, more than 500 million tonnes of agro-industrial by-products and waste are produced, with Brazil contributing 50% of this production, since its agro-industries account for more than 30% of its economy and comprise most of the economic sectors in which the country is internationally competitive, in particular the meat slaughtering and preparation, sugar manufacturing and refining, dairy products, bakery and pasta manufacturing, vegetable oil and juice industries.

Within this context, by-products from the agro-industry can play an important role as a supplement for livestock in Brazil, as they are produced locally, thus avoiding the price of freight as with other traditional foods, since they have a reasonable nutrient composition and are widely available to producers in areas where agro-industries are installed.

The aim of this study was to assess the effect of replacing maize with tomato residue in the diet of laying quails on the physical qualities of the egg.

SUMMARY

A large volume of by-products and agro-industrial waste of good nutritional quality could be used in animal feed, thus reducing production costs.

The aim of this study was to assess the effect of different levels of tomato by-product (TS) on the physical quality of eggs fed to Japanese quails (Coturnix coturnix japonica). 120 birds were housed in a conventional shed with galvanised wire cages and movable side curtains.

The experimental design was entirely randomised, with four treatments and five replicates containing six birds per cage. The treatments consisted of a reference diet, based on maize and soya meal, and three rations with levels of 5, 10 and 15 % ST as a substitute for ground maize. The physical quality characteristics of the eggs were assessed (egg weight, percentage of yolk, albumen and shell, shell thickness, Haugh Unit, yolk index and colour).

The data obtained was subjected to analysis of variance and the means of the significant characteristics were analysed by multiple regression. An increase in egg weight and egg yolk percentage was observed as ST was included in the feed. On the other hand, there was a reduction in the percentage of eggshell with the increase in ST in the feed, however, without altering the thickness of the shell. It was concluded that the levels of tomato by-product evaluated can be used as an alternative ingredient in rations for Japanese quails, improving the physical quality of the eggs.

Keywords: yolk colour, nutritional level, Haugh Unit

SUMMARY

CHAPTER 1

INTRODUCTION

Quail farming is a poultry activity that has been growing in Brazil as part of industrial poultry farming. The quail egg, as a product, is in high demand domestically, and traditional poultry farmers are finding a way to diversify their breeding and supply of eggs to the trade.

In order to maintain and expand this activity, it is necessary to carry out scientific studies to better understand the biology of Japanese quails and thus improve the techniques used, whether in the field of genetics, nutrition, management or reproduction.

The increase in ecological awareness that began at the end of the 20th century has made it clear that humanity's great challenge for the coming decades is to balance the production of goods and services, economic growth, social equality and environmental sustainability (PELIZER; PONTIERI; MORAES, 2007).

In Latin America, more than 500 million tonnes of agro-industrial by-products and waste are produced, with Brazil contributing 50% of this production, since its agro-industries account for more than 30% of its economy and comprise most of the economic sectors in which the country is internationally competitive, in particular the meat slaughtering and preparation, sugar manufacturing and refining, dairy, bakery and pasta manufacturing, vegetable oil and juice industries (ALVES et al., 2007).

Within this context, some by-products from the agro-industry could play an important role in Brazilian poultry feed, as they are produced locally, thus avoiding the price of freight as with other traditional foods, since they have a reasonable nutrient composition and are widely available to producers in areas where agro-industries are installed.

General Objective

To evaluate the effect of using tomato industrial waste in Japanese quail feed on the internal and external quality of the eggs.

Specific Objectives

a) To evaluate the influence of increasing levels of tomato by-product on average egg weight, yolk percentage, albumen percentage, shell percentage and thickness, Haugh Unit, yolk index and yolk colour;
b) To economically determine the level of utilisation of tomato residue in the rations of Japanese quails in production.

CHAPTER 2

LITERATURE REVIEW

Poultry farming

The poultry industry began around 1930, promoting the aggregation of small producers to form large integrated commercial poultry units. These integrated units produced a significant amount of food and consumed industrialised products and feed ingredients, giving rise to supplier and seller companies (MORENG, AVENS, 1990).

The sector is expanding significantly, with an increase in responsibility on the part of the feed industry, since maintaining it implies greater competition. As a result, the industry is investing in researchers in order to find new alternative feed sources that meet the qualitative and economic needs of poultry production (ROSTAGNO et al., 2000).

Alternative foods

According to the author, for a food to fit the alternative or unconventional profile, the indispensable prerequisite is that the input is available in a given region for a minimum period of time and in a quantity that can allow a significant exchange with the conventionally used food (FIALHO; BARBOSA, 1999).

The use of alternative feeds aims to reduce costs in poultry farming at times of the year, or in regions where it is difficult to acquire some of the classic inputs used in animal feed (CUNHA, 2009).

Nascimento et al. (2005) emphasised the contribution of research in order to determine the best options for using alternative energy and protein foods, which should provide good productive and reproductive performance for the birds, reducing feed costs and consequently resulting in greater profitability for the producer.

The use of alternative foods has been constant in rations for broiler chickens and laying hens, but little research has been carried out into quail feeding, considering that these birds have physiological and behavioural differences, differing from the others in terms of feed efficiency and productivity (MURAKAMI; FURLAN, 2002).

With the aim of evaluating the effect of including (0, 5, 10, 15 and 20%) tomato residue (RT) on the productive performance and characteristics of the carcass and main cuts of broiler chickens, Lira et al. (2010) carried out an experiment with 300 male Cobb chicks. The authors concluded that the yields (%) of the cuts were not affected by the use of RT, except for the yields of heart and liver. The use of RT in broiler rations during the period from 1 to 28 days can decrease GP and worsen AC. Tomato residue can be used at levels of up to 20 per cent in broiler feed from 29 to 42 days of age, as this level does not affect weight gain or feed conversion .

An experiment was carried out by Silva et al (2005) to determine the optimum level of inclusion of annatto seed residue (RSU) in broiler feed. They used 1,190 male Ross chickens fed from 1 to 21, 22 to 42 and 43 to 47 days of age with rations containing zero (control), 2.5, 5.0, 7.5, 10.0, 12.5 and 15.0 per cent of MSW. The performance variables evaluated were feed consumption, weight gain and feed conversion in each phase studied. The inclusion of 7.5 per cent MSW improved feed consumption in the period from 22 to 42 days of age, but worsened feed conversion in the total period (1 to 47 days) compared to the control treatment. Excluding the control treatment from the analysis of variance, carcass and thigh yields and thigh weight decreased linearly, while drumstick yield was optimised with the inclusion of 9.9% MSW in the feed. Considering the performance results, the inclusion of up to 5% MSW in broiler feed is recommended.

Tavernari et al (2009) evaluated the effect of including sunflower meal (0, 5, 10, 15 and 20%) in broiler rations to analyse its effects on performance, carcass and cut yields and economic viability. The authors concluded that the addition of 20 per cent sunflower meal to broiler feed up to 42 days of age did not affect the productive performance of the birds.

Cotton farming

Quails originated in North Africa, Europe and Asia and belong to the Fasianidae family (Phasianidae) and the Perdicinidae subfamily, and are therefore from the same family as chickens and partridges (PINTO et al., 2002). The Coturnix coturnix, or European quail, was introduced to Japan in the 11th century. The first writings about this bird date back to the 12th century and record that they were bred for their singing. From 1910 onwards, the Japanese began to study and crossbreed quails from Europe with wild species, obtaining a domesticated type, which came to be called Coturnix coturnix japonica, or domestic quail. They were then exploited for meat and egg production (REIS, 1980).

In Brazil, the Japanese quail was introduced in the 1950s. Although they resemble the wild quails found here, they do not belong to the same family, as the Nothura boraquira (from the Northeast), Nothura minor (from Minas Gerais) and Nothura maculosa (common or partridge) belong to the Tinamidae family (PINTO et al., 2002).

The breeding of laying quails is spreading, favoured by the low initial investment required, the need for small areas to develop the activity and the rapid return on capital (MASSUDA; MURAKAMI, 2008).

According to the AGROPECUARY Census (2012), the quail population totalled 16.4 million, an increase of 5.6% on 2011. The Southeast is the country's largest producer of quails, regardless of whether for meat or egg production. This region accounts for 58.4 per cent of the national figure, with São Paulo being the most important state.

According to Silva et al. (2011), Brazil is the world's fifth largest producer of quail meat and the second largest of eggs, with growth in the country's various regions, with automated farms and new ways of marketing eggs and carcasses.

The current consumer market's demand for quality meat, together with other factors such as rapid animal growth, early production, sexual maturity, high productivity, low initial investment and rapid financial return, make cotton farming a highly promising activity in the country (SILVA; COSTA, 2009).

Oliveira (2007), based on IBGE data, noted that there has been a significant increase in egg production, without major variations in flock size. This increase in productivity can be attributed to the use of technology in the activity, the genetic improvement to which the birds are being subjected and improvements in nutrition, management and health applied to the farms.

According to the same authors, only 21 per cent of producers use alternative feeds such as sorghum to replace traditional feeds. However, 68% of producers use some kind of additive in their feed, such as acidifiers or pro-biotics, which indicates a trend towards better use of feed through the application of nutritional concepts. The feed used on the farms comes from co-operatives or is manufactured on the farms themselves, with 47% of the farmers having their own feed factory that relies on technical support from nutrition companies.

In general, few studies have been carried out on this tomato residue in poultry farming and in the literature researched, no studies were found that used tomato residue in quail feed. It is known that the metabolisable energy values are 1,760 kcal/kg (NRC, 1971, apud JAFARI et al., 2006); 3000 kcal/kg of true metabolisable energy for roosters (Pens Junior, Viola, 1998); 1950 kcal/kg for broilers (SILVA, QUEIROZ, 2002).

In poultry farming, feed accounts for an average of 65 to 70 per cent of production costs. Measures such as replacing conventional products like corn and soya with alternative feed ingredients have been a way of reducing feed costs (TOGASHI; SOARES; MURAKAMI, 2008).

Quail egg consumption and production

Quail breeding in the north of the country is small compared to other regions, representing a total of 0.54 per cent of the herd (IBGE, 2012).

According to data presented by the same research body, in 2012 there was an increase in the number of quails in the Northern Region of around 9.21 per cent when compared to 2011, generating an increase in egg production of 6.26 per cent. Only the states of Acre, Amazonas, Pará and Tocantins were counted for the region in question. When compared to the previous year, the state of Acre had the highest percentage of production (45.16 per cent), followed by the state of Pará, with a small increase of 0.98 per cent.

In the state of Rondônia, there are small breeders producing eggs, which meet the demand of the local population. However, according to IBGE researchers, the data generated by these enterprises is not representative of quail numbers and production when compared to other states, and is therefore omitted by the agency.

Considering egg production in the period 2009/2010, the data shows that 232.398 million dozen eggs were produced in Brazil, representing a significant increase of 20.80%. The states with the highest egg production were São Paulo (59.30 per cent) and Espírito Santo (9.80 per cent), the latter having seen its share fall compared to 2009 (IBGE, 2010).

According to the Brazilian Association of Bars and Shops (2013), the annual per capita consumption of quail eggs by Brazilians was just 14 eggs in 2013 (Figure 1), which is a low figure when compared to the consumption of chicken eggs, which was estimated at 162.59 units/year or 9.76 kilos/year.

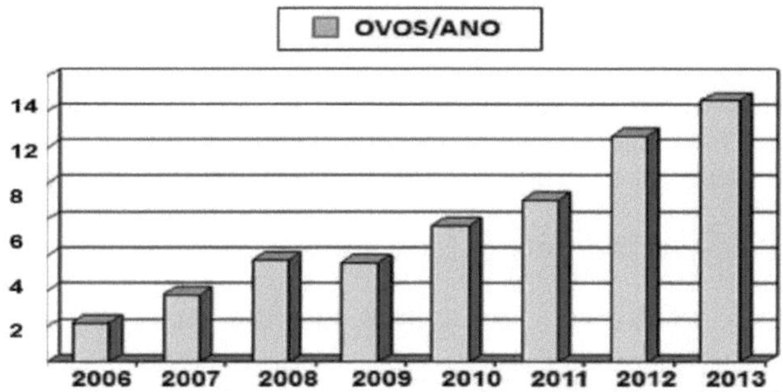

Figure 1 - Annual per capita consumption of quail eggs (Source: IBGE, 2010)

For a long time, eggs were considered a major enemy of healthy eating because they are a great source of cholesterol. However, more recent studies have revealed that ready-made cholesterol (consumed via diet) has an influence of no more than 5% on the rise in total cholesterol in the body of healthy people. This discovery has changed the concept of egg consumption among the American Cardiology Society and has restored eggs' healthiness as a natural alternative to a balanced diet (RADCLIFFE, 2004).

One egg contains around six grams of protein and provides 12 per cent of the daily requirement for this nutrient. It is therefore a source of protein and can help increase lean mass in people who exercise. It has a mix of saturated fats (3.1g - 37.4%) and a mix of monounsaturated fats (3.8g - 46%) and polyunsaturated fats (1.4g - 16.5%), which represent 62.5% of good fats. It also contains fat-soluble vitamins (A, D, E, K) and water-soluble vitamins (thiamine, riboflavin, niacin, choline, folic acid, vitamin B12, biotin), carotenoids (lutein and zeaxanthin), as well as minerals such as iron, zinc and selenium. One quail egg has 70 calories, promoting satiety (ENDRIUKAITE, 2014).

Egg characteristics

The quail egg is normally oval-rounded in shape. Approximately 3 cm long and 2.5 cm wide, it can be approximately one fifth the size of a chicken egg, ranging from 7 to 15 g, with an average weight of 10 g for the Japanese quail. In general, the quail egg represents 6% of body weight, while the chicken egg corresponds to 3% (Table 1), indicating that the quail is more efficient in egg production (ROSTAGNO et al, 2007).

The eggshell is composed of a matrix made up of proteins and interstitial calcified crystals, in a ratio of 1:50. The mineral part is made up of 98.2% calcium carbonate; 0.9% magnesium carbonate; and 0.9% calcium phosphate (Table 2). The organic matrix contains protein (STADELMAN; COTTERILL et al, 1977).

The albumen surrounds the yolk and has the function of absorbing impact, as well as being a source of nutrients. The albumen is made up of a liquid layer surrounding the yolk, a dense middle layer and an outer layer close to the shell, which is similar in composition to the innermost layer (SOUZA SOARES; SIEWERDT et al, 2005).

The yolk consists of a solution of particles in a protein suspension. There are several proteins present in the yolk. Vitellin complexes with lipids to form lipovitellin, and phosvitin is a non-lipid phosphoprotein. The yolk is made up of approximately 65.5 per cent triglycerides, 28.3 per cent phospholipids and 5.2 per cent cholesterol. The amount of carbohydrates in the yolk is around 1.0%. The yolk acquires water from the albumen during the egg storage period, so its moisture content can vary from 46 to 59%, depending on the time and storage conditions (ORDÓNEZ,2005).

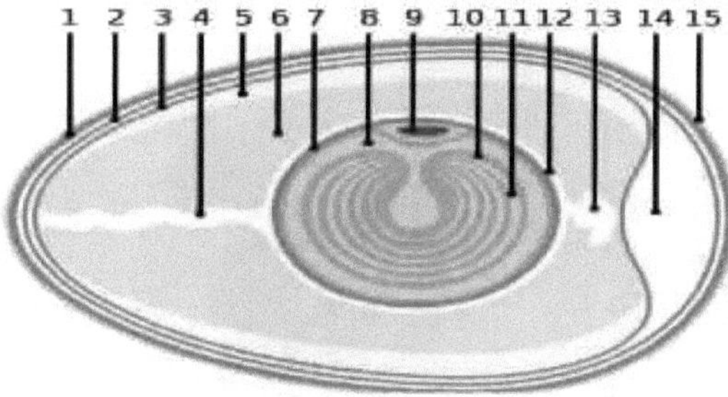

Figure 2 - Egg structure.
Source: http://pt.wikipedia.org/wiki/Ovo
1 - Conch or shell
2 - Outer membrane
3 - Inner membrane
4 - Calaza
5 - External albumin
6 - Medium or clear albumin
7 - Yolk membrane
8 - Centre
9 - Germ
10 - Yellow yolk
11 - White yolk
12 - Albumin inside
13 - Calaza
14 - Air chamber
15 - Conch or shell

The reproductive system of birds consists of ovaries and oviducts. Only the left ovary is functional in the hen and is shaped like a grape cluster, while the right ovary is atrophied (SISSON; GROSSMAN, 1986). (Figures 3,4,5).

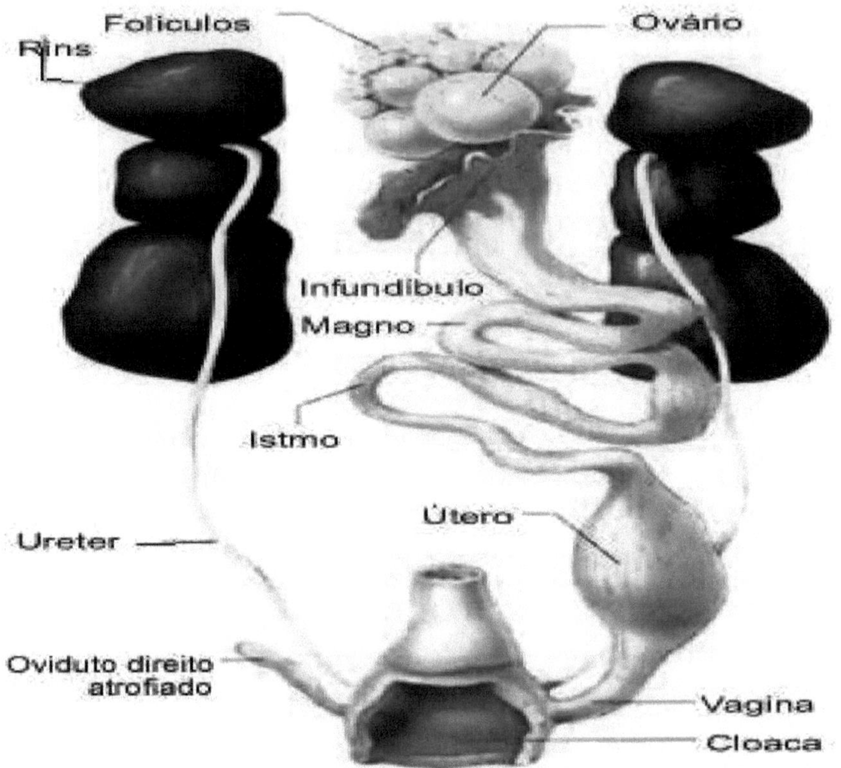

Figura 3 - The female reproductive system has an atrophied right oviduct and ovary.
Source:http://www.mundoeducacao.com/biologia/reproducao-das-aves.htm

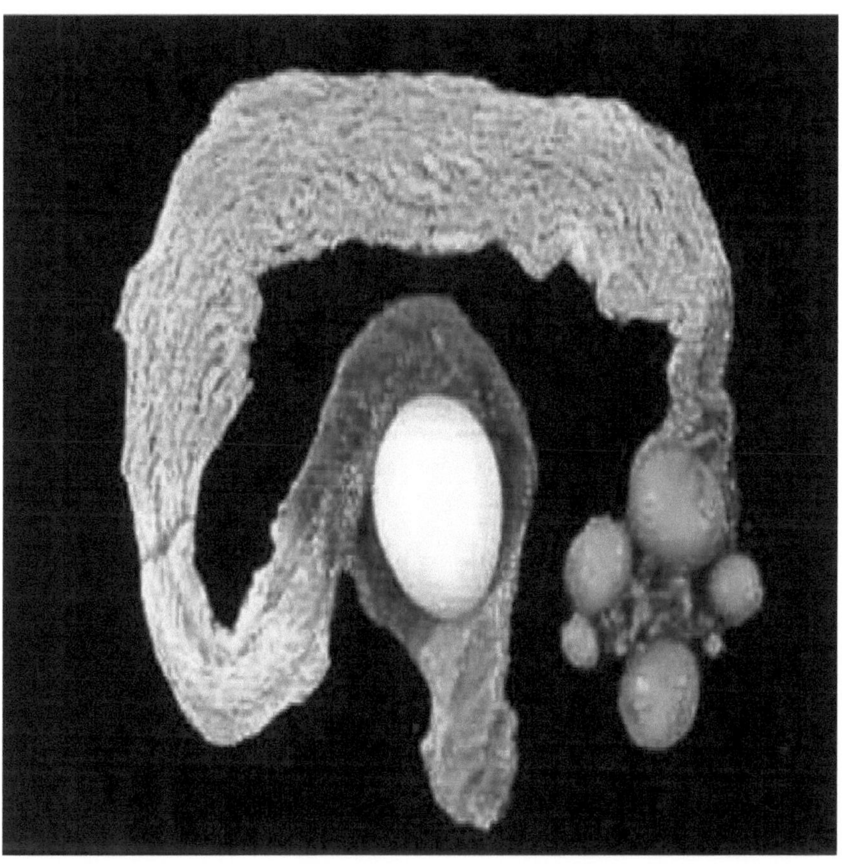

Figura 4 - Reproductive apparatus of a domestic chicken, with an egg formed in the uterus and several eggs in the ovary.

Source: (SISSON; GROSSMAN, 1986).

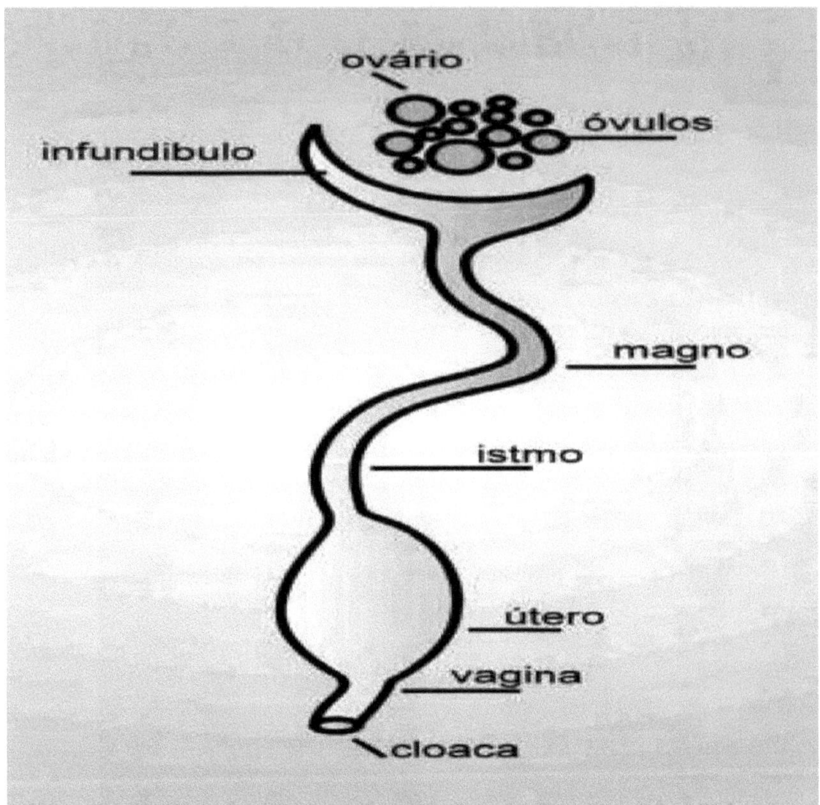

Figure 5 - The oviduct consists of 5 regions: infundibulum, magnum, isthmus, uterus and vagina (SISSON ; GROSSMAN, 1986). **Source:** Geordano Dalmédico 2003

In the infundibulum, fertilisation takes place for 15 minutes, if the eggs are to be reproduced, otherwise this process doesn't take place. In the region known as the magnum, the egg white is formed over a period of three hours, i.e. the various layers of albumen are deposited around the yolk. More than half of the egg's protein content is concentrated in the albumen.

In the region of the isthmus, the inner and outer membranes of the egg are added for approximately 1 hour. Shell formation takes place in the uterus (20/23 hours), when the calcium circulating in the bloodstream is deposited after being secreted by the oviduct's calciferous glands, forming a characteristic crystalline structure.

The shell accounts for 9-12% of the egg's total weight, depending on its size. It takes 15 minutes for the egg to pass through the cloaca, serving only as an internal transit to the external environment (SISSON; GROSSMAN, 1986).

Tomato by-product

A species of Andean origin, the tomato is botanically called Lycopersicon esculentum Mill, a herbaceous solanaceous plant with a wide adaptive capacity. Tomatoes are consumed in fresh and industrialised form by all peoples and their fruit has a high nutritional value (CATI, 1997).

Nutritionally, tomatoes are made up of approximately 94.5 per cent water and are a source of vitamins A, C and E, minerals such as potassium, phosphorus and calcium, carotenoids (lycopene and p-carotene) and phenolic compounds (DUMAS et al., 2003).

Tomatoes are one of the most widespread oilseeds and are grown in the most diverse geographical latitudes. In 2011, world production was 159.02 million tonnes, with China (30.55%), India (10.58%) and the United States of America (7.94%) being the main producers, accounting for around 49% of world production (FAO, 2014). According to the FAO, Brazil is the world's eighth largest producer - it produced 4.42 million tonnes in 2011, in an area of 69.31 thousand ha, with an estimated productivity of 63.85%. Ton/ha, contributing 2.8 per cent of world production. The main producing state was Goiás, followed by São Paulo and Minas Gerais.

According to Pessini (2003), the tomato is probably the best known and most widely consumed vegetable in the world, due to its many uses in human food. As such, the generation of waste from the tomato industry is quite significant, which has led researchers to study alternatives that make it feasible to use tomato by-product (TS) in animal feed, this by-product being used mainly to feed ruminants (AMMERMAN et al., 1963; OJETA;TORREALBA, 2001).

The tomato by-product is made up of: the fruit, the skin of the fruit, the fibrous fraction of the pulp and the seed, considering that the percentage of each component can vary according to the type of fruit processing. Processing consists of pasteurisation (80°C), grinding and pressing, which generates between 20.5% and 42% of the fruit's weight in waste, depending on the processing used (RIBEIRO et al., 2000).

The tomato by-product comes from the tomato pulp or juice industry, which generates approximately 8.1% of the fresh weight in waste, basically made up of seeds and peels, with a small amount of pulp. The proportion of each fraction varies according to the end product, i.e. if it is a peeled product, the residue will be rich in peels, whereas when "Ketchup" or tomato sauce is produced, there is a greater presence of seeds in the residue (OJEDA; TORREALBA, 2001).

For every tonne of tomato extract, spicy sauce or ketchup produced, there is approximately 420, 205 and 230 kg of waste, respectively. It's worth noting that a medium-sized industry receives around 120 tonnes of tomatoes a day (BERTOL; LUDKE; BELLAVER, 2001).

When it leaves the industry, this by-product has a high moisture content, which can exceed 85% (COUTINHO, 1990), limiting its use in natura. However, this high moisture content is due to its processing in the industry, where it passes through extractors and refiners. A lipid content of over 5% can be found in ST (ECKHARDT et al., 2008).

The chemical composition of the tomato by-product can be seen in Table 1. Due to its high fibre content, this ingredient can be classified as a roughage. It has a high crude protein content and is a good source of lysine (13% more than soya meal) and B vitamins. However, much of the protein may be unavailable for use by the animal, given that the tomato undergoes heat treatment during the pulping process.

To produce tomato paste, the fruit is pasteurised (80°C), ground and pressed (FONDEVILA et al., 1994).

Tomato by-product in poultry feed

Nutritional strategies aimed at improving the cost, composition and quality of animal products destined to feed the population are a link between animal production, food technology and the nutrition of the human population (BARRETO et al., 2006).

The use of alternative ingredients aims to reduce the costs of raising poultry at certain times of the year, or in regions where it is difficult to acquire some of the classic inputs used in animal feed (CUNHA, 2009).

Nascimento et al. (2005) emphasised the contribution of research in order to determine the best alternative energy and protein feed options, which could provide good productive and reproductive performance for the birds, reducing feed costs and consequently resulting in greater profitability for the producer.

The use of alternative ingredients has been constant in feed for broilers and laying hens, but little research has been done on quail feed, considering that these birds have physiological and behavioural differences, differing from others in terms of feed efficiency and productivity (MURAKAMI; FURLAN, 2002).

With the aim of evaluating the effect of including tomato by-product (TS) (0, 5, 10, 15 and 20 per cent) on the productive performance and characteristics of the carcass and the main cuts of broiler chickens, Lira et al. (2010) carried out an experiment with 300 male chicks. The authors concluded that the yields of the cuts were not affected by the use of ST, except for the yields of heart and liver. The use of ST in broiler feed during the period from 1 to 28 days of age can reduce weight gain (WG) and worsen feed conversion (FC). However, tomato by-products can be used at levels of up to 20% in broiler feed from 29 to 42 days of age, without harming the GP and FC of the birds.

According to literature data, it is known that the metabolisable energy values of tomato by-products are 2,806 kcal/kg of metabolisable energy for layers (LOUREIRO et al., 2006); 3,000 kcal/kg of true metabolisable energy for roosters and 1,950 kcal/kg for broilers (PENS JUNIOR; VIOLA, 1998), 2006); 3,000 kcal/kg of true metabolisable energy for roosters and 1,950 kcal/kg for broilers (PENS JUNIOR; VIOLA, 1998); 2,351 kcal/kg for chicks between 1 and 8 days old and 2,465 kcal/kg for chickens between 10 and 17 days old (LIRA et al., 2011).

Experiments have been carried out with different levels of tomato by-product inclusion for commercial layers, and the results found by these researchers point to a maximum level of 15 per cent inclusion in the diet of layers, without affecting the productive parameters in the laying of these birds (YANNAKOPOULOS et al.,1992; DOTAS et al.,1999).

According to Persia et al. (2003), seeds from tomato processing were used in an experiment with broiler chickens from 8 to 21 days of age, including levels of up to 20 per cent of the ingredient in corn and soya meal-based rations and found that using up to 15 per cent did not interfere with the birds' performance when compared to the reference ration, even promoting an improvement in the pigmentation of the birds' carcasses.

According to Loureiro et al. (2007), tomato bran caused a decrease in yolk weight and percentage, however, up to 15% inclusion, heavier yolks were obtained when compared to the reference feed. According to this study, tomato bran can be used as an alternative ingredient in rations for commercial layers.

Work carried out with Japanese quails showed that the inclusion of 5 per cent tomato pulp (the main source of lycopene) in the diet had an antioxidant effect, while the addition of 10 per cent had a pro-oxidant effect (BOTSOGLOU et al., 2004).

CHAPTER 3

MATERIAL AND METHODS

Experiment site

The study was conducted at the facilities of the Coturnicultura Sector of the Experimental Centre of the Camilo Castelo Branco University, UNICASTELO, Descalvado-SP campus, from August to October 2012. The laboratory analyses were carried out at the Animal Nutrition and Biogeochemistry Laboratory of UNICASTELO, Descalvado-SP campus.

Processing the tomato by-product

100kg of tomato extract by-product was obtained from Indústria Predilecta, located in the district of São Lourenço do Turvo in the city of Matão/SP (Figures 6 and 7).

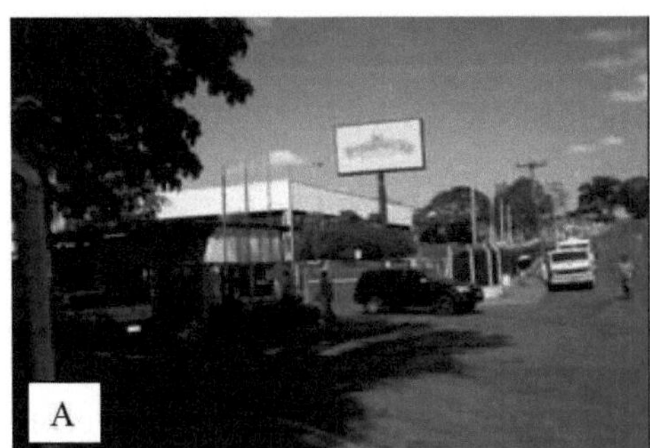

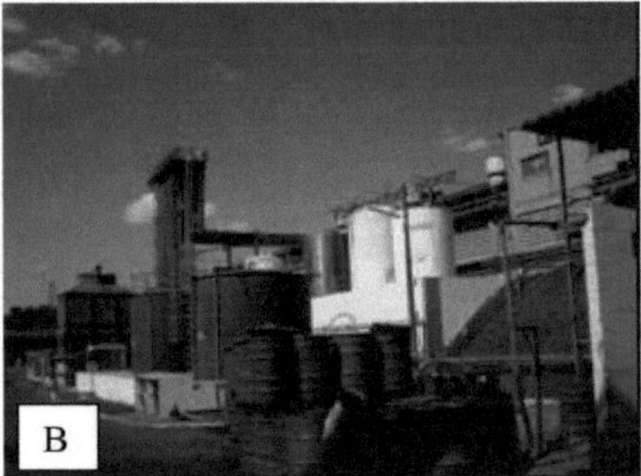

Figure 6 - External view of Predilecta, Matão-SP (Source: Personal archive, 2012)

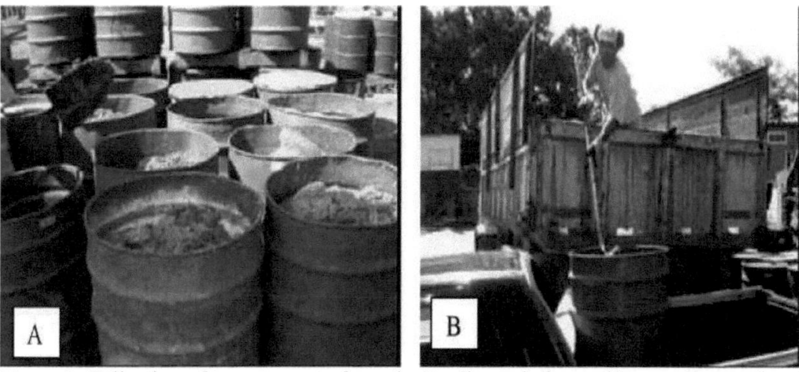

Figure 7. Collection of tomato waste from the Preditecta industry (Source: Personal archive, 2012).

Firstly, the tomato by-product was dried in the open air in the shade, laid out evenly on a plastic tarpaulin until the moisture was completely removed (Figure 8), then ground in a hammer mill with a 5 mm sieve (Figure 9).

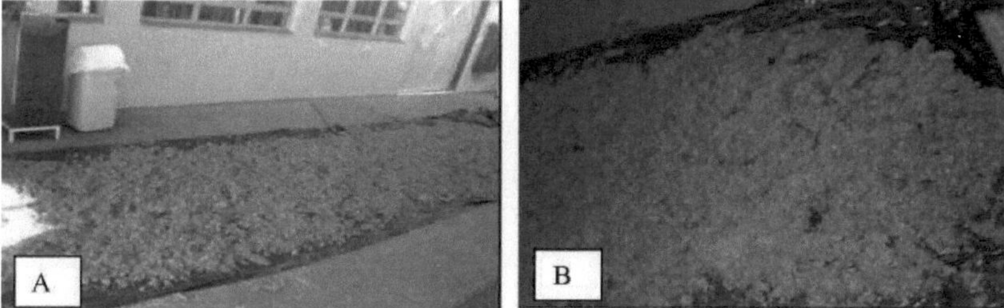

Figure 8. Drying tomato waste in the open air (Source: Personal archive, 2012).

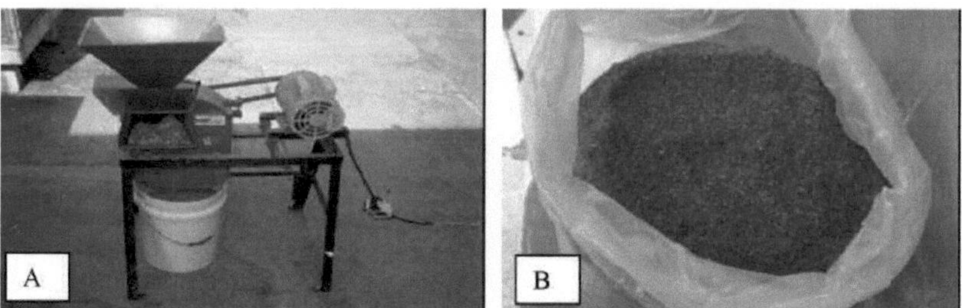

Figure 9. Grinding tomato waste after drying in open air (Source: Personal archive, 2012).

Subsequently, the tomato by-product was sampled and the samples were dried in an oven with forced air circulation at 55° C for 72 hours and ground in a Thomas-Willey type mill fitted with sieves with a 1 mm mesh opening.

Table 1 - Chemical composition of the tomato by-product.

Nutrient (%)	Average	Minimum	Maximum
Dry Matter	20,4	6,5	35,0
Crude Protein	19,2	10,4	26,0
Ether extract	12,1	2,7	19,0
NDF	29,9	51,6	68,6
FDA	45,9	38,8	28,5
NDT	59,7	46,5	72,5
Calcium	0,3	0,2	0,6
Phosphorus	0,5	0,4	0,9

NDF=Neutral detergent fibre; FDA=Acid detergent fibre; NDT=Total digestible nutrients.

Source: Campos (2005)

Animals and experimental design

A total of 120 Japanese quails (Coturnixcoturnixjaponica) were used, initially aged 35 days and with an average weight of 126.18 ± 1.56 grams. They were housed in a conventional shed (6.0 x 4.0 metres) with galvanised wire cages arranged in a single row with trough-type feeders and nipple-type drinkers.

The quails were vaccinated at seven days of age against NewCastle disease and infectious bronchitis. Artificial lighting was provided using 100-watt incandescent bulbs in a 16-hour light programme during the productive phase.

The birds were distributed in a completely randomised experimental design, with four treatments and five replicates with six birds per experimental unit.

The treatments consisted of a reference ration based on maize and soya meal and three rations with levels of 5, 10 and 15% tomato by-product as a substitute for maize. The centesimal and calculated composition of the rations can be found in Table 1 and 2, according to Silva and Costa (2009).

Table 2. Centesimal and calculated composition of rations with different levels of tomato by-product for laying Japanese quails.

Ingredients	Tomato by-product			
	T0%	T5%	T10%	T15 %
Grain maize	63,52	59,24	54,96	50,52
Soya meal - 45%	20,40	21,40	22,40	25,24
Tomato residue[1]	0,00	5,00	10,00	15,00
Calcitic limestone	6,56	6,52	6,48	6,48
Bicalcium phosphate	1,60	1,64	1,68	1,68
Protenose	7,52	5,80	4,08	0,68
Mineral and vitamin supplements[2]	0,40	0,40	0,40	0,40
TOTAL	100,00	100,0 0	100,00	100,00
Calculated chemical composition				
ME (kcal/kg)	2.570	2.570	2.570	2.570
Crude Protein (%)	19,10	19,10	19,13	19,15
Calcium (%)	3,15	3,15	3,12	3,12
Total phosphorus (%)	0,40	0,41	0,43	0,43
Total lysine (%)	1,20	1,20	1,20	1,20
Total methionine (%)	0,47	0,47	0,47	0,47
Met+cist total (%)	0,80	0,80	0,80	0,80
Sodium (%)	0,20	0,20	0,21	0,21
Chlorine (%)	0,26	0,25	0,25	0,24
Potassium (%)	0,82	0,81	0,80	0,80
BED3 (mEq/kg)	221,78	221,72	221,68	221,7 0

1. Composition of the tomato industrial waste used (Predilecta): 96.69% DM; 18.78% PB; 63.12% FDN; 43.77% FDA; 17.92% Cellulose; 25.85% Lignin.
2. Composition of the mineral and vitamin supplement (kg of product): Vitamin A (min)12,000.00 IU/kg; vitamin B1 (min) 2.40mg/kg; vitamin B12 (min) 20.00 mcg/kg; vitamin B2(min)11.00mg/kg, vitamin B6(min) 4.00mg/kg ; vitamin D3 (min) 2,400.00 IU/kg vitamin E(min) 24.000 IU/kg; vitamin k3 (min)3.00mg/kg; cobalt (min) 0.18mg/kg; copper (min) 9.00mg/kg; iron (min) 45.00mg/kg; iodine (min) 0.90 mg/kg; manganese (min) 54.00mg/kg selenium (min) 0.32 mg/kg; sodium (min)1.800.00 mg/kg; zinc (min) 45.00mg/kg; folic acid (min) 2.00 mg/kg; pantothenic acid (min)19.95mg/kg; biotin (min) 0.14 mg/kg; niacin (min) 48.00mg/kg; choline (min)180.00 mg/kg;
3. Dietary Electrolyte Balance (Mongin, 1981) = [(%Na*10,000/22.990) + (%K*10,000/39.102)] - (% Cl*10,000/35.453).

Table 3. Composition of the tomato by-product used from the Predilecta company.

Nutrient (%)	Average
MS	96,69
PB	18,78
NDF	63,12
FDA	43,77
Cellulose	17,92
Lignin	25,85

DM = Dry Matter; PB= Crude Protein; FDN= Neutral Detergent Fibre; FDA= Acid Detergent Fibre.

Water and feed were given freely throughout the experimental period, with food being distributed twice a day at 8am and 5pm.

Methods for analysing egg quality

The egg characteristics assessed were: egg weight, yolk, albumen and shell percentages, shell thickness, Haugh Unit, yolk index and yolk colour.

The average egg weight was obtained by weighing all the intact eggs produced in each treatment replicate on a precision scale (x = 0.01g) during the last three days of each 21-day period.

After total weighing, three eggs per repetition were taken at random to assess the internal and external quality of the eggs. Each egg was weighed individually and placed in trays duly identified by the repetitions. They were broken on a flat surface to measure albumen height, yolk colour, yolk height and diameter, using a digital caliper. Yolk colour was obtained according to the Roche® colorimetric range, on a scale of values from 1 to 15.

The yolks were weighed individually on a precision scale to measure their respective percentages in relation to the weight of the total egg. The weight of the albumen was obtained by subtracting the yolk and shell from the total weight of the egg.

The height of the albumen was used to estimate, together with the weight of the egg, the Haugh Unit (HU) characteristic. The Haugh Unit is a measure of albumen quality. The formula described by Brant and Shrader (1958) was used to calculate the HU:

$$UH = 100 \log (H + 7.57 - 1.7\ W^{0'37})$$

Where H = albumen height (mm); W = egg weight (g); 7.57= correction factor for albumen height; 1.7= correction factor for egg weight.

The yolk index was obtained from the ratio between the height and diameter of the yolk (NESHEIM et al., 1979).

The height and diameter of the yolk were obtained using a digital caliper, after the albumen had been completely removed from the egg.

The eggshells were washed in running water to remove any excess albumen and kept in suitably labelled trays to dry at room temperature for 48 hours. After drying, the shells were weighed to calculate the percentage of shell in relation to the total weight of the egg.

After weighing them, they were used to measure the thickness of the shell in millimetres using a digital caliper, taking three measurements in the equatorial zone of the egg to obtain an average per sample unit.

Statistical Analysis

The data obtained was submitted to analysis of variance and the means of the significant characteristics were analysed by multiple regression and orthogonal contrast, at 5% significance, using the statistical software SAS (Version 9.0, SasI nstitute Inc., Cary, NC, USA).

CHAPTER 4

RESULTS AND DISCUSSION

The average values for the percentage of eggs laid, feed consumption and the external and internal quality characteristics of the eggs are shown in Tables 3, 4 and 5.

There was an effect of the treatments ($p<0.05$) on the average egg weight, yolk percentage and shell percentage (Table 3). The tomato residue linearly influenced egg weight and yolk percentage as the residue was included in the diets, showing an increase in the respective values (egg weight = 10.75972+0.05788*X (R^2=0.87) - Figure 6; yolk percentage = 31.30812+0.15952*X (R^2=0.85) - Figure 7). On the other hand, there was a linear reduction in the percentage of eggshell as the tomato residue in the birds' diets increased (shell percentage = 13.47467-0.05321*X (R2=0.62) - Figure 8). However, no difference was observed in the percentage of albumen and eggshell thickness during the evaluation period.

Table 4 - Average values[1] of egg weight and its proportions (yolk, albumen and shell) and eggshell thickness of Japanese quails fed a ration containing increasing levels of tomato by-product.

Waste Tomato (%)	Egg weight (g)	Yolk (%)	Bark (%)	Bark thickness (mm)
0	10,67±0,88 b b	31,06±3,62	13,59±1,69 a	0,260±0,056
5	11,21±0,78 a a	32,42±3,90	12,99±1,80 b	0,253±0,056
10	11,25±0,78 a a	32.96±3.97	13,20±1,63 b	0,257±0,046
15	11,64±0,79 a a	33,55±4,13	12,20±1,96 b	0,261±0,057

P-value	0,045*	0,029*	0,036	0,136
CV (%)	8,54	9,07	12,21	14,85

1.Mean ± standard deviation; *Linear effect ($p<0.05$); *Egg weight (g) = 10.75972+0.05788*X (R^2=0.87); Yolk (%)=31.30812+0.15952*X(R^2=0.85); Shell (%)= 13.47467-0.05321*X (R^2=0.62); Letters different column, differ significantly by orthogonal contrast ($p<0.05$)

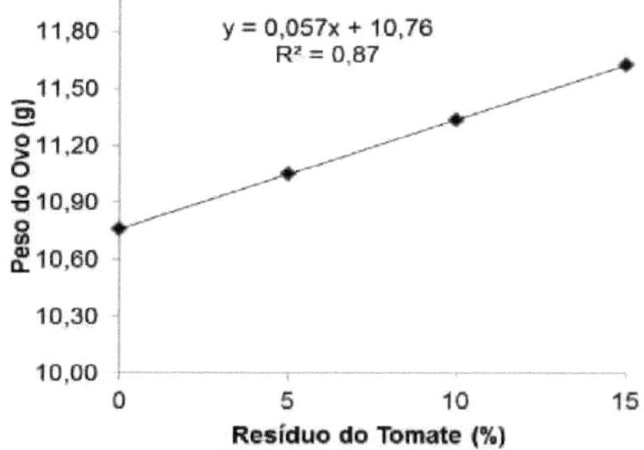

Figura 10. Average egg weight values of quails fed containing different levels of tomato residue.

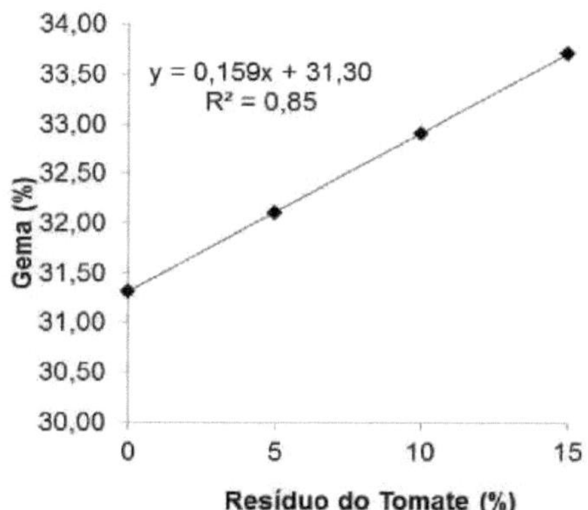

Figura 11. Average values of egg yolk percentage of quails fed diets with different levels of tomato residue.

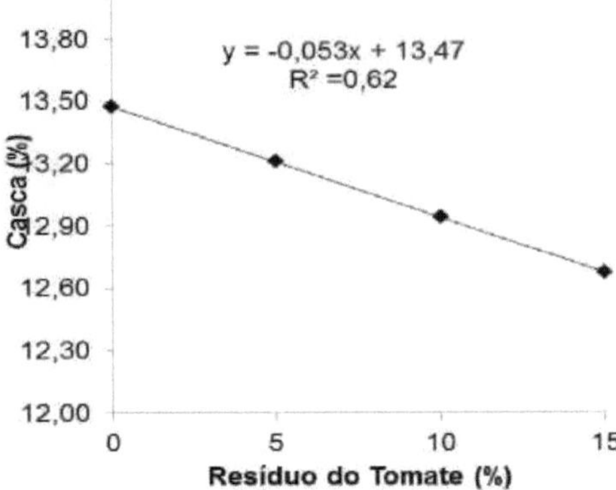

Figura 12. Average values for eggshell percentage in quails fed diets containing different levels of tomato residue.

Studies with laying hens fed diets containing up to 20% tomato bran found no effect of the treatments on average egg weight (DOTAS et al., 1999; LOUREIRO et al., 2007). These same authors observed a decrease in the percentage of yolk as the inclusion of tomato by-products in the birds' diets increased, justifying a possible increase in fibre in the diets, negatively interfering with the absorption of other nutrients.

With regard to eggshell thickness, the results observed corroborate those of Dotas, Zamanidis and Balios (1999), who found that the use of up to 12% tomato bran in the feed of laying hens did not lead to differences in eggshell thickness when compared to those birds fed corn and soya meal-based feed.

The increase in egg weight as the tomato by-product was included in the birds' feed did not show the same behaviour for the percentage of eggs laid, as can be seen in Table 4. Among the treatments with the different levels of ST, there was no difference in egg laying, although it was lower than that of the control treatment (without tomato meal). There was no difference in the average daily feed consumption for birds in all treatments.

Table 5 - Average values[1] of egg-laying percentage and daily feed consumption (grams/bird) of Japanese quails fed a diet containing tomato by-products.

Tomato residue (%)	Posture (%)	RAC (g/bird/day)
0	72,61 ± 1,40 a	28,65 ± 1,95
5	66,93 ± 3,09 b	25,96 ± 1,03
10	63,96 ± 3,01 b	25,12 ± 1,25
15	68,57 ± 3,30 b	27,45 ± 1,36
P-value	0,052	0,256
CV (%)	9,56	11,25

1. mean ± standard deviation; different letters in the column differ statistically by orthogonal contrast (p<0.05)

Table 5 shows the average values for the internal quality characteristics of the eggs. There were no significant differences (p>0.05) for the characteristics HU, yolk index and yolk colour.

Table 6 - Average values[1] of the egg quality characteristics of Japanese quails fed rations containing tomato by-products.

Tomato waste (%)	Unit Haugh	Yolk index	Colour of Gem[2]
0	90,32±4,56	0,49±0,04	6,47±1,06
5	90,06±4,36	0,50±0,06	6,27±1,26
10	91,16±3,83	0,47±0,05	6,25±1,00
15	90,64±4,60	0,46±0,05	5,95±0,91
P-value	0,341	0,628	0,290
CV (%)	4,22	27,58	17,43

1 - Mean ± standard deviation; *Linear effect (p<0.05); Different letters in the column differ significantly by orthogonal contrast (p<0.05); 2 - Roche colourimetric range® (scale from 1 to 15)

The results for the yolk index characteristic were above the recommended ideal (between 0.39 and 0.45) for classification as good quality (EISEN; BOHRE; MCKEAN, 1962). With regard to the colour of the yolk, contrary to what was expected from the natural pigment present in tomatoes to increase the colour of the yolk, the lycopene in the residue may have been oxidised during processing (drying and grinding) and thus did not differentiate the colour of the egg yolk.

The same was not found in the studies carried out by Yannakopoulos, Tserveni and Christaki (1992), in which they evaluated levels of 0, 8 and 15% inclusion of tomato bran in laying hen rations and found better colour in the yolk of laying hen eggs.

CHAPTER 5

CONCLUSION

Under the conditions of this study, tomato residue can be used as an alternative ingredient in production quail rations at an inclusion level of 15 per cent, without affecting egg quality.

BIBLIOGRAPHICAL REFERENCES

ALVES, A.C. N.; MATTOS, W.R.S.; SANTOS, F.A.P. et al.Partial replacement of maize silage by dehydrated maize gluten meal in the diet of lactating Holstein cows. **Revista Brasileira de Zootecnia**, 36 (5): 1590-1596, 2007.

AMMERMAN, C.B.; ARRINTON, L.R.; EPLOGGINS, P. Nutritive value of Dried tomato pulp for ruminants. **Agricultural Food Chemistry**, 11 (4): 347- 349 1963.

BRAZILIAN ASSOCIATION OF BARS AND RESTAURANTS. Available at http://www.abrasel.com.br/index.php/atualidade/noticias/2010. Accessed on 13 Feb. 2014.

BARRETO, S.C.S.; ZAPATA, J.F.F.; FREITAS, E.R. et al. Fatty Acids from the
yolk and egg composition of layers fed diets containing coconut bran. **Pesquisa Agropecuaria Brasileira**, 41 (12): 1767-1773, 2006.

BOTSOGLOU, N.; PAPAGEORGIOU, G.; NIKOLAKAKIS, I. et al. Effect of Dietary Dried Tomato Pulp on Oxidative Stability ofJapanese Quail Meat.
Journal of Agriculture land Food Chemistry, 52: 2982-2988, 2004.

BERTOL, T.M.; LUDKE, J.V.; BELLAVER, C. Effect of finishing pig weight at the beginning of feed restriction on performance and carcass quality. **Revista Brasileira de Zootecnia**, 30: 417-424, 2001.

BRANT, A.W.; SHRADER, H.L. **Equipment and methods for measuring egg quality.** Washington: Department of Agriculture, 1958,17p.

CATI - Coordination of Integral Technical Assistance. **Technical manual of crops** 2 ed. Campinas; CATI, p 125-132, 1997.

CAMPOS, W. E. **Evaluation of industrial tomato residue in broiler chicken feed**. Belo Horizonte: UFMG Veterinary School, 2005. 123p. (Doctoral thesis).

COUTINHO, L.L. Nutrient replenishers. In: REUNIÃO ANUAL DA SOCIEDADE BRASILEIRA DE ZOOTECNIA,1990, Campinas, SP. **Annals...** Campinas: SBZ, 1990. p.617- 632.

CUNHA, F.S.A. **Evaluation of cassava (**Manihotes culenta Crantz**) and by-products in quail** (Coturni xJaponica) **feed**. 2009. 98p Thesis (Integrated doctorate in zootechnics: Area of concentration:

Production of non-ruminants) - Federal Rural University of Pernambuco Recefe, PE.

DOTAS, D. S.; ZAMANIDIS, S.; BALIOS, J. Effect of dried tomato pulp on the performance and egg traits of laying hens. **British Poultry Science.** 40: 695- 697, 1999.

DUMAS, Y. M; DADOMO, G.D. LUCCA et al. Effects of environmental factors and agricultural techniques on antioxidant content of tomatoes. **Journal of the Science of Food and Agriculture**, 83: 369-382,2003.

ECKHARDT, O.H.O.; HORTA, F.C.; MORETTI, A.S. et al.Initiatives of the pork agro-industrial system to signal excellence. **Revista Pork World**, Campinas, 46: 156-162, 2008.

EISEN, E.J.;BOHRE, B.B.;MCKEAN, H.E. The Haugh Unit as a measure of egg albumen quality**. Poultry Science**, 41: 1461-1468, 1962.

ENDRIUKAITE.L.**The egg fulfils 12% of daily needs.** INDUSTRIAL POULTRY FARMING. Available at: http: //www.aviculturaindustrial.com.br>Accessed on 05 April. 2014.

FAO - Food and Agriculture Organisation of the United Nations. Available at: <http://www.faostat.fao.org>. Accessed on 30 January 2014.

FONDEVILA, M.; GUADA, J. A.; GASA, J. et al. Tomato pomace as a protein supplement for growing lambs. **Small Ruminant Research**,13 (1): 117-126, 1994.

BRAZILIAN INSTITUTE OF GEOGRAPHY AND STATISTICS. **Production of Municipal Livestock**: 2010. Rio de Janeiro, v.38, 65p. 2011 Available at: <http://ibge.gov.br/produc-o-da-pecuaria-municipal-2010-v-38-brasil.html>. Accessed on: 08 January 2014.

IBGE. BRAZILIAN INSTITUTE OF GEOGRAPHY AND STATISTICS. **Municipal Livestock Production 2012**. Available at: < http: www.ibge.gov.br> Accessed on 29 January 2014.

LIRA, R.C; RABELLO.C.B.V; SILVA E.P. et al. Chemical composition and energy values of guava and tomato residues for broilers at different ages. **Revista Brasileira de Zootecnia,** 40 (5): 10191024, 2011

LIRA, R.C; RABELLO, C.B.V.; LUDKE, M.C.M.M. et al. Productive Performance of broiler chickens fed tomato waste. **Revista Brasileira de Zootecnia**, 39 (5): 1074-1081, 2010.

LOUREIRO, R.R.S.; RABELLO, C.B.V.; LUDKE, J.V. et al. Tomato bran (Lycopersicum esculentum Mill.) in the diet of commercial layers. **Acta Scientiarum Animal Science**, 29 (4): 387-394, 2007.

LOUREIRO, R.R.S.; RABELLO, C.B.V.; DUTRA JR., W.M. et al. Metabolisable energy values and apparent metabolisation coefficients of dry matter and crude energy of tomato bran for commercial layers, In: REUNIÃO ANUAL DA SOCIEDADE BRASILEIRA DE ZOOTECNIA, 43, 2006, João Pessoa. **Proceedings...** João Pessoa: SBZ 2006 (CD-ROM).

MASSUDA, E. M.; MURAKAMI, A. E. Cost of production in cotton farming - laying farms. **PUBVET**, 2 (36): 31- 37, 2008.

MONGIN, P. Recent advances in dietary anion-cation balance: application in poultry. **Procedure Nutrition Society**, 40:285-294, 1981.

MURAKAMI, A.E.; FURLAN, A.C. Research into the nutrition and feeding of laying quails in Brazil. In: SIMPÓSIO INTERNACIONAL DE COTURNICULTURA, 1., 2002, Lavras, MG. **Proceedings...** Lavras: Federal University of Lavras, 2002. p.113-120.

NASCIMENTO, G. A. J.; COSTA, F. G. P.; AMARANTE JÚNIOR, V. S. et al. Effects of Replacing Maize with Cassava Scraps in the Feeding of Broiler Chickens during the Fattening and Final Stages. **Revista Ciência e Agrotecnologia**, 29 (1): 200-207, 2005.

NESHEIM, M.C.; AUSTIC, R.E.; CARD, L.E. **Poultry Production.** 12[th]ed., Philadelphia, USA: Lea and Febiger, 1979, p 288-289.

ORDÓNEZ, J.A. Eggs and derived products. In:Food technology. Foods of animal origin. Porto Alegre: Artmed, 2005. p. 269-279.

OJEDA, A.; TORREALBA, N. Chemical characterisation and digestibility of

tomato process ingresidues in sheep. **Cuban Journal Agricultural Science**, 35 (4): 309-312, 2001.

OLIVEIRA, B. L. Management in automated farms for commercial laying quails. In: SIMPÓSIO INTERNACIONAL DE COTURNICULTURA, 3, 2007, Lavras. **Proceedings...** Lavras: Federal University of Lavras, 2007.p 232.

PELIZER, L.H.; PONTIERI, M.H.; MORAES, I.O. Utilisation of Agro-Waste

Industrial Biotechnological Processes as a Perspective for Reducing Environmental Impact. **Journal of Technology Management & Innovation,** 2: 118-127, 2007.

PENZ JÚNIOR, A.M.; VIOLA, E.S. Nutrition. In: SOBESTIANSKY,J.; WENTZ, I.; SILVEIRA, P.R.S.; SESTI, L.A.C. (Ed.). **Intensive pig**

farming: production, management and herd health. Concórdia: EMBRAPA, 1998. p 45- 60.

PERSIA, M.E; McCAY, C.M.; SMITH, S.E. et al. Nutritional evaluation of dried tomato seeds. **Poultry Science**, 82 (1): 141-146, 2003.

PINTO, R.; FERREIRA, A. S.; ALBINO, L. F. T. et al. Protein and energy levels for laying Japanese quails. **Revista Brasileira de Zootecnia**, 31 (4): 1761-1770, 2002.

PESSINI, M. M. O. **Residues of acetamiprid and thiamethoxam in staked tomato (Lycopersicones culentummill.), in different modalities of application**. 2003. p 88. Dissertation (Master's in Animal Sciences) - **Escola Superior de Agricultura "Luiz de Queiroz" da** Universidade de São Paulo, ESALQ, Piracicaba, São Paulo.

RADCLIFFE, J.S. The importance of pork carcass modifiers for meat quality. **Porkworld**, Campinas, v. 22, p. 50-54, 2004.

REIS, L. F. S. D. **Quails, breeding and exploitation.** Lisbon: Agros, 1980. 222p.

RIBEIRO, A. C.; RIBEIRO,S. D. A.; ANTONIO, M. S. et al. Composition chemistry of different tomato agro-industry residues destined for animal feed. In: REUNIÃO ANUAL DA SOCIEDADE BRASILEIRA DE ZOOTECNIA, 37, 2000, Viçosa, MG. **Anais...** Viçosa: UFV, 2000. (CD Rom).

ROSTAGNO, H.S.; BUNZEN, S.; ALBINO, L.F.T. et al. Methodological advances in feed evaluation and nutritional requirements for poultry and pigs. In: 44th Annual Meeting of the Brazilian Society of Animal Science...**Proceedings**, p.295-304. Jaboticabal, SP. 2007.

SILVA, J.H.V.; COSTA, F.G.P. **Table for Japanese and European quails Jaboticabal**, SP:Funep, 2009, p.67-78.

SILVA. J.H.V.;JORDÃO FILHO.J.; COSTA, F.G.P. et al. Nutritional requirements of quails. In: XXI BRAZILIAN CONGRESS OF ZOOTECNIA. 21, 2011. Maceió, AL. **Proceedings...** Maceió: Federal

University of Alagoas, 2011, (CD-Rom).

SOARES, L.A.; SIEWERDT, F. Poultry and eggs. Pelotas: Editora da Universidade UFPEL, 2005. 137 p.

SISSON, S.; GROSSMAN, J.D. **Anatomy of domestic animals**. Rio de Janeiro: Guanabara Koogan, 1986. 2v.

TOGASHI, C.K.; SOARES, N.M.; MURAKAMI, A.E. Technical survey of quail egg producing farms located in Bastos and region, State of São Paulo. **Informações Econômicas**, 38 (12): 28-30, 2008.

YANNAKOPOULOS, A.L.; TSERVENI-GOUSI, A.S.; CHRISTAKI, E.V.
Effects of locally produced tomato meal on the performance and egg quality of laying hens. **Animal Feed Science and Technology**, 36 (1): 5357,1992.

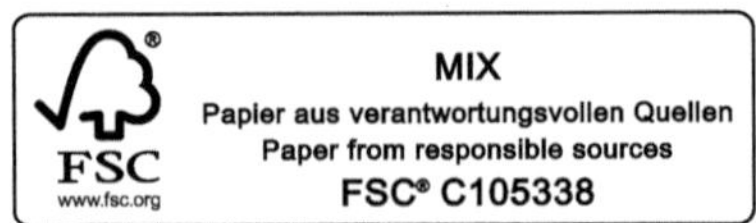

Printed by Books on Demand GmbH, Norderstedt / Germany